Table of Contents

Introduction

The Pritikin Diet is basically a healthy diet. Pritikin didn't start as a weight loss program -- it started as a way to reverse heart disease, high blood pressure, diabetes, says Dr. James Kenney, chief nutritionist of the Pritikin Longevity Center. "What makes eating healthy in America difficult is that most restaurant foods -- particularly fast restaurant food is designed to make people fat and sick. So popular did the low-fat craze become that in 1992 the U.S. Department of Agriculture introduced its much-vaunted food pyramid guidelines that recommended Americans lay off the fat and load up on grains and cereals, which are carbohydrates. But there was a problem. During the 1990s, despite the new guidelines and the glut of low-fat and fat-free products available, Americans got even fatter. While most experts agree that Americans' increasingly sedentary lifestyle and fondness for fast food contributed to the nation's growing girth, others postulate that the low-fat label misled consumers into believing that such products contained fewer calories, causing them to eat even more. The low-fat message was interpreted as if you had a product that was lower in fat it was good for you without thinking of calories," says Professor Marion Nestle of New York University's Department of Nutrition, Food Studies and Public Health. "The best example is the Snackwell phenomenon: Snackwell cookies were advertised as low-fat cookies but they had almost the same number of calories." Nutritionists also note that in order to make products low-fat, companies had to replace the fat with something else usually carbohydrates. Enter Dr. Atkins and the low-carb diet craze currently sweeping the nation. Whereas low-fat diets like Pritikin and Ornish warned followers against eating high-fat foods like steak and eggs, Atkins followers avoided the carbohydrates that are the mainstay of a low-fat lifestyle. Not surprisingly, low-carb diets have come under attack by everyone from low-fat diet proponents to scientists and the media. In Diet Wars, Talbot speaks with science journalist Gary Taubes, who wrote a controversial article for The New York Times Magazine that questioned whether the food pyramid was wrong and limiting carbohydrates was the way to go. I got crucified in a variety of publications, Taubes tells frontline. A Washington Post reporter went after me, the Center for Science in the Public Interest went after me because suddenly I turned around and said, 'Maybe low-fat diets don't work and maybe low-carbohydrate diets are the answer. Taubes admits to being surprised by the ferocity with which his article was attacked. "People are more polarized on this than they are in politics," he says. "I'm stunned. What most nutritionists and industry experts do agree on is the fact that America is facing an obesity problem of epidemic proportions. This is the public health issue of our generation," says Dr. James Hill, director of the University of Colorado's Center for Human Nutrition. When you see 65 percent of Americans are overweight or obese, what amazes me is that anyone maintains a healthy weight in this environment. The Pritikin diet was developed by the late Nathan Pritikin, a self-trained scientist who sparked much controversy during the 1970s and early 1980s with his claims about the link between diet and heart disease. Since Pritikin's death, he has been vindicated, with many studies confirming his claims.You are right that we all need some fat in our diet. Furthermore, a recent study indicated that if an individual were to follow a low-fat diet, such as that recommended by the American Heart Association (less than 30 percent of calories from fat), his or her life would be prolonged by only a few months. One might conclude, in your words, ``why bother. This requires a little closer consideration, however. First, according to Pritikin principles, a 30 percent fat free diet is too high in fat to show substantial health benefits. The Pritikin program suggests a maximum of 10 percent fat.

Definition

The Pritikin diet is a low calorie, high bulk, low fat and low cholesterol diet. Diet generally eat foods that have an average of less than ten percent of daily calories from fat. It is almost entirely vegetarian, and those who adhere to this diet avoid processed and fatty foods.

History

Nathan Pritikin, the originator of the Pritikin Diet was diagnosed with heart disease at the age of 42. In the late 1950s when Pritikin was diagnosed, about 40% of calories in the average American diet came from fats. Pritikin was given little medical guidance on how lifestyle changes might slow his heart disease. Although educated as an engineer, Pritikin devised his own heart-healthy diet, which he followed rigorously. Based on his experience, he opened the Pritikin Longevity Center in Florida in 1975. Here people could come and immerse themselves for one or more weeks in the Pritikin Eating Plan. Nathan Pritikin developed cancer and committed suicide in 1985 at the age of 69. At his autopsy, doctors discovered no signs of heart disease, a fact they attributed to his rigorous life-long adherence to his diet. Robert Pritikin, Nathan's son, took over the Longevity Center enterprises after Nathan's death. While maintaining the core of the original diet, Robert updated some of the concepts in his book The Pritikin Principle: The Calorie Density Solution. published in 2000. According to Nathan Pritikin", "All I'm trying to do is wipe out heart disease, diabetes, and obesity." That would be a miracle for anyone to complete, being as these three diseases are the three major killers of Americans. Nathan Pritikin had a passion for both research and a desire to cure himself of his heart disease. He developed a low-fat, low-cholesterol, high-carbohydrate diet, which he credits for saving his life. Pritikin's cholesterol fell below the safe 150 mg/dL to approximately 100 mg/dL. This happened, after eliminating all animal products from his diet. His research led him to the conclusion that most illnesses seen in older patients were not due to the natural inevitable consequence of aging, but due to diets. Diets rich in saturated fats and animal products. His desire was to not only treat his own heart disease but also to eradicate typical Western illnesses caused by the rich Western diet. Michael Greger M.D shares the story of his grandmother, who inspired him to go into medicine:

Description

At the time Pritikin developed his diet, his concepts seemed quite radical. However Pritikin was ahead of his time, and today, despite a few controversies, most of his principles have been incorporated into advice given on how to reduce the risk of developing cardiovascular disease by mainstream organizations such as the American Heart Association. The Pritikin Plan is a diet that is high in whole grains and dietary fiber, low in cholesterol, and very low in fats. Fewer than 10% of calories come from fats. This is much lower than the average twenty-first century American diet, in which about 35% of calories come from fats. It is about half the amount of fats recommended in the federal Dietary Guidelines for Americans 2005. The diet is also lower in protein than suggested in the federal guidelines. However, in general, the Pritikin Plan reflects many recommendations in the Dietary Guidelines for Americans 2005. It results in low calorie, nutritionally balanced meals. In addition, the Pritikin plan calls for 45 minutes daily of moderate exercise such as walking, another recommendation in line with mainstream medical advice. The newest version of the Pritikin Plan calls for avoiding foods that are calorie dense. These are foods that pack a lot of calories into a small volume of food (e.g. oils, cookies, cream cheese). Instead, Plan followers are encouraged to choose low-calorie foods that provide a lot of bulk (e.g. broccoli, carrots, dried beans). This way, dieters can eat a lot of food and feel full without taking in a lot of calories. The plan does not limit the amount of healthy fruits and vegetables a dieter can eat, and it suggests that dieters divide their food among five or six smaller meals during the day. The Pritikin Plan is based on eating a particular number of servings of each group of foods as follows:

• At least five ½-cup servings of whole grains such as wheat, oats, and brown rice or starch vegetables such as potatoes, and dried beans and peas. Refined grain products (white flour, regular pasta, white rice) are limited to two servings daily, with complete elimination of refined grain products considered optimal.

• At least four 1-cup servings of raw vegetables or ½-cup servings of cooked vegetables. Dark green, leafy, and orange or yellow vegetables are preferred.

• At least three servings of fruit, one of which can be fruit juice.

• Two servings of calcium-rich foods such as nonfat milk, nonfat yogurt or fortified and enriched soymilk.

• No more than one 3.5 cooked serving of animal protein. Fish and shellfish are preferred. Lean poultry should optimally be limited to once a week and lean beef to once a month. This diet is easily adapted to vegetarians by replacing animal protein with protein from soy products, beans, or lentils.

• No more than one caffeinated drinks daily. Instead drink water, low-sodium vegetable juices, grain-based coffee substitutes (e.g. Postum) or caffeine-free teas.

• No more than four alcoholic drinks per week for women and no more than seven for men, with red wine preferred over beer or distilled spirits.

• No more than seven egg whites per week

• No more than 2 ounces (about 1/4 cup of nuts) daily

• Other foods such as unsaturated oils, refined sweeteners (e.g. Concentrated fruit juice, corn syrup), high-sodium condiments (e.g. Soy sauce), and artificial sweeteners (e.g. Splenda) are "caution" foods. They are not recommended, but if they are used, the plan gives guidance in how to limit them to reasonable amounts. Animal fats, processed meat, dairy products not made with non-rat milk, egg yolks, salty snacks, cakes, cookies, fried foods and similar high-calorie choices are forbidden.

The Plan also calls for at least 45 minutes of moderate exercise daily such as walking. People who check into the Longevity Center receive a personalized exercise program after a physician gives them an examination. This doctor follows their progress while at the center and makes a written report at the end of their stay that they can take home to their personal physician. People who do not visit the Longevity Center can receive support and inspiration through the Plan's extensive Web site. Pritikin has also developed a Family Plan aimed at families with obese children.

Pritikin Meal Plan

Week One

- Day One Start Eating Right

- Day Two Lower Blood Pressure

- Day Three Healthy Sandwiches

- Day Four Big Salads For Weight Loss

- Day Five Eat Less Meat & Lower Cholesterol

- Day Six Healthy Comfort Food

- Day Seven Snack Smarter

Week Two

Shopping List for Week Two

- Day Eight Bison: The Better Red Meat

- Day Nine Feast On Fish

- Day Ten Veggie-Rich Soups

- Day Eleven Eat Beans, Shed Fat

- Day Twelve Go For Whole Grains

- Day Thirteen Potatoes Are Good For You!

- Day Fourteen Enjoy Fruit, Not Juice

Foods that are allowed when starting the Pritikin Diet

Vegetables

According to the Pritikin website, people starting the Pritikin Diet are encouraged to consume five or more servings of fresh vegetables each day. On the program, a serving is defined as 1/2 cup of cooked vegetables or 1 cup raw. No vegetables are off-limits, though canned vegetables are discouraged because of their high sodium content. Followers are instructed to aim for a variety of colors of vegetables daily, particularly red, dark green, yellow and orange vegetables.

Carbohydrates

The diet allows five or more 1/2-cup servings of whole grains each day. This can be legumes, beans, high-starch vegetables such as winter squash or potatoes, or whole grains like brown rice, quinoa, whole wheat or oats. The Pritikin Diet strongly recommends avoiding refined carbohydrates like white rice and pasta or bread prepared from white flour.

Fruit

When you start the Pritikin Diet, plan on having four or more servings of fresh fruit daily. The only restrictions on your fruit consumption are to limit yourself to 2 ounces of avocados daily and to choose whole fruit over fruit juice whenever possible. A single serving of fruit is enough to fit in the palm of your hand.

Dairy Products

You can have two servings of high-calcium, non-fat dairy products per day, choosing from 1 cup of non-fat regular or soy milk, 1/2 cup of non-fat ricotta cheese or 3/4 cup of non-fat yogurt. You should avoid whole- and low-fat dairy items and try to use low-sodium brands of cheese whenever possible. Followers of the plan are also told to avoid whole eggs in favor of no more than one or two egg whites consumed daily.

Nuts and Seeds

Nuts and seeds like sunflower seeds, peanuts, macadamia nuts, almonds, cashews and pumpkin seeds are allowed on the Pritikin Diet, but it's recommended that you eat only about 1 ounce per day. The Pritikin website advises against eating coconuts more than once a month because of their high fat content.

Protein

The Pritikin Diet allows much less protein than many other diet programs: dieters are instructed to consume only one 3.5-ounce serving of animal-based protein like lean red meat, lean poultry, fish or seafood each day. When you start the diet, you're encouraged to eat one serving of beans, legumes or soy products such as tofu per day instead of animal protein. If you want to eat meat, you're advised to try to eat red meat only once a month and poultry no more than once a week.

Beverages

You can drink herbal tea, coffee substitutes made from powdered roasted grains and bottled, tap or mineral water on the Pritikin Diet. You can also use up to 2 tablespoons of cocoa powder daily and drink three 8-ounce cups of caffeinated tea or one 8-ounce cup of caffeinated coffee per day. Women can have no more than four alcoholic beverages weekly, while men can have seven. Wine -- especially red wine is recommended over beer or liquor.

Function

Unlike many diets, the Pritikin Plan never claims that a person will lose a certain amount of weight within a certain length of time. People who follow the Plan, which is a low calorie diet, do lose weight and keep it off so long as they stay on the plan. However, the Plan is primarily intended to cause changes in lifestyle that will promote heart health for a lifetime.

Precautions

As with any diet, people should discuss with their physician the pros and cons of the Pritikin Plan based on their individual circumstances. This diet may not be right for actively growing children.

Risks

The greatest risk to this diet is that it is too rigorous for many people, and that they will lose weight on the diet and then gain it back, causing weight cycling (yo-yo dieting) and the potential health problems that repeated weight gain and loss cause.

The Pritikin Principle: Short-Term and Long-Term Effects

Daniel says that adopting the diet changes suggested by the Pritikin Principle would certainly cause improvements in the short run for people switching from a standard American diet. "But in the long run, extreme low-fat diets create many problems, not the least of which is the fact that most people can't stay on them. Those with enough willpower to stick with them are highly likely to develop health problems including low energy, inability to concentrate, depression, immune system breakdown, and even weight gain," warns Daniel. Says Kimball, "Like most diet plans, there are some good things to take from the Pritikin Principle, but there is no substitute for educating yourself about nutrition and making good choices that you can live with for a lifetime.

Everyone who's ever thought about going on a diet has at least heard of The Pritikin Approach: a low-fat diet, not vegetarian, but largely based on vegetables, grains and fruits. Fat in the diet accounts for a mere 10%. Since 1976, more than 70,000 people have spent time at the Pritikin Longevity Centers learning how to eat healthy, prepare low-fat meals and snacks, and incorporate exercise and stress-reduction techniques into their lives. Several books by Nathan Pritikin carried the message of the Pritikin approach to the masses. It was an approach designed largely to promote well-being by lowering cholesterol and helping diabetics normalize their blood sugar without taking insulin. That people lost weight was an added plus.

The Pritikin Principle: What You Can Eat

Some foods have more calories packed in them, bite for bite and pound for pound, claims Pritikin. If we eat foods with fewer calories per pound, we can fill up on these foods and still have the kind of calorie deficit that we need to lose weight. Pritikin doesn't shy away from the basic principle that weight loss is achieved by eating fewer calories than you burn each day, which is refreshing, given the spate of current diet books that attempt to ignore that simple but unalterable axiom. The Pritikin Principle has more than 20 pages of charts listing the caloric density of all kinds of foods, from snacks to sausages, listing them in calories per pound to graphically demonstrate the striking calorie differences between low-density foods and high-density foods. Not surprisingly, the more processed the food, the more likely they are packed full of calories. Corn, for instance, starts out at a somewhat reasonable 490 calories per pound. By the time it ends up in a tortilla chip at your favorite Mexican restaurant, it's skyrocketed to 2,450 calories per pound. However, eat it with guacamole, and the combination (avocado dip with the chips) drops the number to 1,450 calories per pound. The plan is to eat food with a large volume of fiber and water to fill up your stomach vegetables, fruits, beans, and natural, unprocessed grains. These foods, he claims, "create tremendous feelings of fullness, or satiety, in your stomach." In addition to eating three meals a day, the program incorporates two "calorically light" snacks as well. While Pritikin doesn't have you counting calories, you do have to possess a basic understanding of how to calculate the "average caloric density of your meal," and then keep that average below a certain number. Exercise is strongly recommended, and walking is his favorite. How much is just right to maintain weight loss? Based on observations of obese people who lost weight and kept it off, Pritikin suggests "All of us should use 30 miles a week as a goal." For the rest of us, however, he suggests one 30-minute walk a day. Going at a good clip, you might average 12 to 15 miles a week.

The Pritikin Principle: How It Works

To lose weight, most of us will need to keep the average caloric density of each meal below 400 calories per pound. Since most vegetables fall below 200 calories per pound, when they are eaten with meat and starches, they bring down the calorie average of each meal. High-carbohydrate food, along with pasta and hot cereals, range between 230 to 630 calories per pound. Animal protein goes from 400 calories per pound (some fish) to 1,400 (that juicy porterhouse steak) to 2,170 (bacon). By combining the leanest portions of animal protein with plenty of vegetables, you can get the caloric density down to a level where you will lose weight, according to Pritikin's plan. To keep within the suggested guidelines, Pritikin suggests we eat whole, unprocessed, and natural carbohydrate-rich foods, such as grains, vegetables, and fruit. Those preferred are:

• Brown rice

• Millet

• Barley

• Oats

• A wide assortment of dark green lettuces

• Onions

• Potatoes

• Squash

• Beans (black turtle beans, chickpeas, lentils, lima and pinto beans)

• Apples

• Pears

• Strawberries

• Bananas

Some processed whole-grain foods, such as oatmeal, are acceptable. Even white-flour pasta is okay, as long as it is combined with vegetables to bring down the caloric density of the whole meal.

Other guidelines: Eat small portions of lean beef, chicken, and low-fat dairy products. Fish is fine, preferably three servings per week of omega-3 rich seafood. Avoid fried foods, dressing with fat, and fatty sauces. Eat frequently. Have three meals a day plus two snacks. Stay active and avoid salty foods. Artificial sweeteners such as Splenda are okay. And decaf tea, once frowned upon, is fine. The book contains several pages of suggested meals and tips on how they might be improved with substitutions, as well as a restaurant guide for everything from a Junior Bacon Cheeseburger at Wendy's to buttered noodles in a French restaurant to a serving of almond chicken in a Chinese establishment. More than 50 recipes are also included.

The Pritikin Principle: What the Experts Say

There seems to be little dispute that you will lose weight on the Pritikin diet or that it is generally a nutritionally rich diet low in calories. But there are caveats: "Because fat makes one feel full, the extremely low fat content of this diet will make those following it often feel hungry," says Teryl L. Tanaka, RD, the clinical nutrition manager at the Santa Monica UCLA Medical Center. Consequently, she adds, the likelihood is high of the weight returning after one stops strictly adhering to the diet. James Hill, PhD, the director of the Center for Human Nutrition at the University of Colorado Health Sciences Center in Denver, agrees that the diet is not practical for many people. While observing that people staying at the Pritikin Centers do really well losing weight, he asks: "How realistic is the diet once they get away from the centers and into the real world. Both the Pritikin diet and the nutritionally similar Ornish diet are extremely low in fat, Hill notes, down to 10% of total calories. "Yes, if we could do that we would all be healthier, but it is very hard to follow that formula in our environment," he cautions. "It's difficult to maintain such a low-fat content of our diets if you eat out often, and it takes time to prepare good,-tasting low-fat food. Most people do not have the time to spend hours each day preparing food. Another problem, adds Tanaka, is that the low-fat content may actually be harmful to our health, "Pritikin also inhibits the intake and absorption of fat soluble vitamins, and can even limit the amount of essential fatty acids provided by the diet needed for normal cell function, healthy skin and tissue, growth and development."

The Pritikin Principle: Food for Thought

What do most nutritionists and health authorities like about the diet? Its strict limit of animal products -- often associated with a variety of major diseases -- and that it incorporates exercise and stress reduction, along with overall low calorie intake. But this is qualified with a concern that the extremely low-fat regimen is difficult to stick with over the long haul.

Other guidelines:

• You can eat small portions of lean beef, chicken, and low-fat dairy products.

• Fish is fine, preferably three servings per week of salmon or other fish rich in omega-3 fatty acids.

• Avoid fried foods, dressing with fat, and fatty sauces.

• Eat three meals a day plus two snacks.

• Stay active and avoid salty foods.

• Artificial sweeteners are OK on the plan, too.

Stops Snoring and Sleep Apnea

About 40 million Americans suffer chronic health issues related to long-term sleep deprivation. At Pritikin, physicians who are experts in sleep evaluation and treatment help guests stop storing and/or get control of other sleep-robbers, like sleep apnea. The result for many has been the return to a long, restful night's sleep, and stunning improvement in well being

Arthritis Pain Relief

Aching, throbbing, sharp pain. However you describe it, arthritis hurts. As yet, there's no cure for the disease, but recent research has found that lifestyle changes can significantly lessen pain and discomfort. Of particular benefit is losing excess weight, regular exercise, and relaxation training. All are hallmarks of the Pritikin Program.

Arthritis Pain Relief

Stop Smoking

You'll be immersed in a customized program to optimize success. Pritikin is the ideal place to quit smoking. You're free of familiar triggers, and your healthy new lifestyle will help keep weight in check. "Pritikin should be sold out on its smoking program alone," says Pritikin alum and ex-smoker Charles Krobot. "I know of no other program where people can stop smoking and lose weight at the same time."

Stress Management

Everyone wants more happiness and less stress. Working with psychologists, you will learn how to maximize your stress hardiness, cope with high-risk situations, make the most of relationships, fend off the blues, and more. "I used to think that everyone, as they got older, got sadder, sicker, and more troubled," says Pritikin alum Monty Preiser. "But with Pritikin, I've realized life really can be fun again."

Reduce Cancer Risk

Many cancers, including epidemic ones like lung, breast, and prostate, are linked to the way we live. Lifestyle factors like controlling weight, avoiding tobacco, eating healthfully, and exercising regularly offer powerful means of reducing risk. Recently, for example, scientists at UCLA discovered in lab settings that the Pritikin Program actually induced prostate and breast cancer cells to die.

Disease Prevention

A health vacation at the Pritikin Center lays the foundation for a lifetime of good health and disease prevention. You'll lose weight without feeling hungry, regain your vitality, and feel healthier, stronger. Now's your chance. Says Pritikin alum Linda Stempel, "I look and feel better now, at age 60, than I did at age 30. Pritikin is all about possibilities. It's all about what you can have in life."

Family Health

Our child obesity epidemic has been described by the U.S. Surgeon General as "the terror within." Researchers predict that today's kids may be the first generation in America in which parents outlive their children. The Pritikin Family Program, held every summer, teaches children how to grow into lean, healthy adults. And the entire family learns how fun and doable healthy living can be.

Men's Health

Now is the time to get clean. Give yourself optimal protectionagainst a heart attack, stroke, diabetes, prostate cancer, and even impotence. Live a happier, more balanced life. With Pritikin, it's easy. There's no calorie counting, no food points, no special foods you have to buy. And once you see and feel the benefits, you'll kick yourself for not getting started sooner.

Women's Health

The first step in managing your health is knowing who your enemy is. The disease many women fear most is cancer, but the disease that kills more U.S. women than any other is heart disease. At Pritikin, you'll learn how to protect yourself from heart disease and related conditions, including weight gain. And you'll discover that middle age and the post-menopause years can be a time of getting healthier, not older.

Healthy Mind-Healthy Body

You're excited, you're motivated, you're seeing results with Pritikin living. Now, how do you stay motivated? Many alumni return regularly for health vacations at Pritikin. Laughs Fil Warihay, age 74 and a size 4, who has vacationed at Pritikin eight times: "I love being the old lady who keeps up with the youngsters." For developing a lifelong love affair with healthy living, here are some tips.

• Focus on natural foods and lots of vegetables and fruit

• Sport is a daily component

• Scientific studies prove positive influence on heart health

• Whole grain products and vegetables provide a lot of healthy fiber

• Low calorie and protein levels can lead to hunger

• Nothing for meat lovers

• Very low-fat content

• Low-salt and low-fat preparation can become monotonous in taste and difficult when eating outdoors.

Calories Points Count

For those who want to lose weight with Pritikin, a daily calorie quantity of 1,000 / 1,200 kcal is recommended. So you can't avoid counting calories here either. The choice of food is also limited and very low in fat. You really don't have to stress about excessively having to count the calories that you eat. It can be a pain to count every calorie, but with this diet, you'll know that the foods you are eating are low calorie.

Sport & Exercise

Sport is an important component of the Pritikin diet. The daily program includes a minimum of 45 minutes of running (jogging, Nordic walking, etc).

Focuses on Healthy Eating

One of the key pros of the Pritikin Principle Diet is that it really focuses on healthy eating. The foods allowed in the diet are foods that are full of great vitamins and minerals. So you really get the important nutrients that help to keep your body healthy. Also, the foods that you eat make you feel full as well, which means you don't constantly have to deal with cravings.

Allows a Variety of Foods

There are a variety of different foods that you are allowed to eat as well. This makes it a better diet than some diets that are extremely restrictive. When you have a variety of foods to eat, you are less likely to get bored.

Starch is Allowed in Moderation

While there are some diets that totally get rid of carbs, this diet allows you to have some carbs as long as it is done in moderation. This is a healthier choice than just totally getting rid of the carbohydrates in your diet.

Nutrient Assessment

The calorie supply of 1,000 kcal per day should not be undercut in any case, because otherwise, it can come to lack of nutrients. Particularly with the demanding, daily sport workload of the Pritikin diet, physical performance can be impaired. The low-fat content impairs the absorption of fat-soluble vitamins (A, E, D, and K) and the low content of meat and dairy products can lead to an insufficient supply of calcium, iron, and zinc.

Exercise For Weight Loss

Due to the rather low-calorie intake of 1,000 kcal per day, a rather rapid weight loss of 1-2 kilos per week can be expected at the beginning, depending on the initial weight. For a healthy weight reduces the number of calories should not be undercut and a weight loss of 0.5 to 1 kilo per week should be aimed at. Weight loss does not happen overnight. It takes a great deal of dedication to lose weight, usually by changing eating habits and exercising regularly. This two-step approach to weight loss may not produce the miraculous effects found in a "magic pill," but it does guarantee long-lasting results. The dietary changes restrict calorie intake while exercising boosts the body's metabolic rate. When used in combination, a calorie-burning effect occurs that leads to weight loss. In general, every exercise routine burns calories; however, aerobic exercises tend to produce the best results. Aerobic Exercise Trumps Resistance Training for Weight and Fat Loss: According to Duke researchers, aerobic exercise trumps resistance training for weight and fat loss. And here are some benefits

• Lowered total cholesterol and LDL or "bad" cholesterol

• Lowered blood pressure, so that people with high blood pressure may no longer need pressure-lowering drugs

• Better control of insulin levels, so that people with type 2 diabetes can often control their disease through diet and without drugs

• Decrease in the circulating levels of compounds that increases the risk of heart disease and blood vessel damage

• A substantially reduced risk of heart disease, hypertension, type 2 diabetes, and breast, colon, and prostate cancers.

• Lifetime freedom from obesity and all of its associated health risks and lifestyle-limiting conditions

Recipe

Turkey Meatloaf

Ingredients

• 1/2 pound turkey (extra lean) ground

• 1/3 cup onions minced

• 1/2 tablespoons garlic minced

• 1/3 cup green bell peppers diced

• 1/3 cup red bell peppers diced

• 1/3 cup carrots diced

• 1/3 cup celery diced

• 1/3 cup Italian parsley chopped

• 3/4 cups oatmeal uncooked

- 1/3 cup whole-wheat bread crumbs (low sodium)

- 2 tablespoons tomato paste no-salt-added

- 1 tablespoon Dijon mustard no-salt-added

- 1 tablespoon Worcestershire sauce

- 1 tablespoon soy sauce, low sodium

- 1/2 tablespoon thyme (fresh) leaves picked

- 1/2 tablespoon black pepper freshly ground

- 1.5 egg whites whipped

- 1 dash Tabasco to taste

- 1/2 cup tomato sauce no-salt-added

Instructions

- Preheat oven to 375 degrees F.

- Use a food processor to grind the turkey.

- Once it's ground, add it to a large mixing bowl.

- One by one, add each ingredient.

- Thoroughly combine all ingredients together.

• Lightly spray a non-stick meatloaf pan.

• Pour the entire turkey mixture into the pan and spread it evenly.

• Cover with aluminum foil and bake for 45 minutes.

• Remove foil and cook for another 25 minutes.

• Remove meatloaf from the oven and allow pan to cool for at least 20 minutes before serving.

Roasted Potato Wedges

Ingredients

• 1 pound potato (Russet) washed and thinly sliced into wedges

• 1/4 cup red wine vinegar

• 1/4 cup water

• 1 teaspoon onion (granulated)

• 1 teaspoon garlic chopped

Instructions

• Preheat oven to 400 degrees F.

• Soak potato wedges in vinegar and water for about 30 minutes.

• On a nonstick baking sheet, spread out wedges. Sprinkle with onion and garlic.

• Bake in oven for about 20 minutes, turning once. Remove from oven when wedges are crispy on both sides.

Garbanzo Chocolate Cookies/Brownies

Ingredients

• 4 cups garbanzo beans cooked (no-salt-added canned beans are fine)

• ½ cup apple puree (ready-made, no-sugar-added apple sauce is fine)

• 2 Tbsp. vanilla extract

• 1½ cups Splenda divided

• 1½ cups Hershey cocoa powder (Unsweetened) OR 1½ cups de-fatted bitter chocolate (melted over water bath)

• ½ cup egg whites

Ingredients For Vanilla Sauce:

• 1 cup Greek yogur (fat-free plain) (or fat-free sour cream)

• ¼ cup Splenda

• 1 Tbsp. vanilla extract

Instructions

• Procedure For Cookies/Brownies:

• Preheat oven to 350 degrees F.

• In a food processor, puree garbanzo beans, apple puree, vanilla, and ½ cup Splenda. Blend until smooth.

• In a small bowl, combine cocoa powder (or melted chocolate) with 1 cup Splenda. If using cocoa powder, combine cocoa powder with Splenda plus just enough warm water to create a thick paste.

• Add cocoa mixture to garbanzo mixture in food processor. Blend until well incorporated.

• Using a whisk or hand blender, whip egg whites until fluffy. Add egg whites to food processor mixture and blend for another 2 minutes.

• For cookies, scoop up dough, one heaping tablespoon at a time, onto a nonstick cookie sheet or a regular sheet lightly sprayed with Pam or lined with parchment paper. For brownies, spread out mixture evenly, just as you would with regular brownie mixture, into an 8" by 8" Pyrex dish or a nonstick cooking tray.

• Bake cookies or brownies at 350 degrees for 25 minutes. For the brownies, the edges should be starting to recede from the sides of the tray. Cool, then cut into 3"x 3" squares.

Pritikin Chicken in Sweet Chili

Ingredients

• 4 ounces chicken breast cleaned

• 1 tablespoon Pritikin All-Purpose Seasoning

• 1/4 cup whole wheat flour (optional)

• 3 tablespoon sweet chilli pepper (crushed)

• 1/4 cup apple juice (concentrated) (or 2 tablespoons of splenda)

• 1 cup hot water

• 1 teaspoon corn starch

- Fresh Salsa

Instructions

- Season chicken breast with all purpose seasoning

- Combine sweet chili pepper, hot water and apple juice concentrate and let sit for 10 minutes.

- Lightly flour chicken breast and sear in a medium hot skillet on both sides

- Pour sweet chili mixture over chicken and cover.

- Lower flame and turn chicken on other side and cook for 8 minutes.

- Mix cornstarch with 2 tablespoons cold water and thicken the pan juices to create sauce.

- Plate with fresh salsa, or chopped tomatoes, onions and cilantro and herbs.

Vegetable Quesadilla

Ingredients

- 2 cups julienned fresh vegetables

- 1 whole-wheat, extra-thin lavash bread

• 3 tablespoons shredded fat-free mozzarella cheese

• 1 tablespoon finely chopped cilantro (optional)

• 2 tablespoons fat-free sour cream, for serving

• 1/4 cup no-salt-added pico de gallo or no-salt-added salsa, such as Enrico's, for serving

Directions

• In a nonstick skillet over medium-high heat, sauté the vegetables until crisp-tender, about 3 minutes. On a warm griddle, place the lavash bread and let the side facing the heat get hot. Turn the bread over on the griddle, and sprinkle the cheese on the top side. On half of the top side, spread the sautéed vegetables and cilantro, if using.

• When the cheese begins to melt, fold the bread in half to cover the vegetables. Press firmly using a tool like a large firm spatula or the bottom of a pan. Flip, cook for about 2 minutes, and press. Remove from the heat. Cut the quesadilla into 4 pieces. Serve 2 pieces per person with fat-free sour cream and pico de gallo on the side.

Ingredients

• 48 ounces chicken breast halves, skinned

• 1 cup chicken stock or 1 cup vegetable stock, minus fat

• 1 cup tomato sauce

Directions

• Place chicken pieces in a large bowl or pan. Place all the remaining ingredients, except yogurt, in a blender, and blend.

• Pour the mixture over the chicken, turning to coat well. Cover and marinate over night in the refrigerator.

• About 1 hour before serving, transfer chicken and marinade to a baking dish. Cover and bake at360 degrees for 50 minutes, or until chicken is nearly done.

Mashed Potatoes With Corn and Fat-Free Sour Cream

Ingredients

• 2 pounds potatoes (Yukon Gold)

• 1 cup corn (fresh) or frozen kernels (thaw if frozen)

- 1/2 cup milk nonfat very hot

- 1/4 cup sour cream, fat free

- Dash nutmeg ground (optional)

Instructions

- Boil potatoes in water until soft (about 25 minutes).

- Meanwhile, in a medium-hot nonstick skillet, sauté corn kernels until soft, about 5 minutes.

- In a food processor, blend corn to a paste-like consistency.

- In a large mixing bowl, mash potatoes using a wire whip. Add corn, hot milk, sour cream, and nutmeg (optional). Whisk until potatoes are fluffy. Serve immediately.

Cornbread

Ingredients

- 1 pound cornmeal

- 1/4 cup flour (stoneground whole-wheat)

- 2 teaspoons baking powder

- 1/4 teaspoon cinnamon ground

- 1/4 teaspoon nutmeg ground

- 2 teaspoons Splenda optional

- 5 cups milk soy or skim

- 2 teaspoons vanilla extract

- 2 cups egg whites

Instructions

- Preheat oven to 350 degrees F.

- In a large bowl, combine all the dry ingredients (cornmeal through Splenda) and mix well. Make a hole in the center and pour in the milk and vanilla. Use a wire whisk to gently mix in the liquids, using a circular motion.

- In a separate bowl, whip egg whites until fluffy. Pour into mixture and mix in.

- Pour mixture into muffin cups or cake tin, and bake in a hot water bath* at 350 degrees for 45 minutes.

- To prepare a water bath for baking, put your filled muffin trays or cake tin in a larger pan and add enough boiling-hot water to reach halfway up the side of the smaller pan.

Ingredients

• 1 pound meat substitute

• 1 cup bread crumbs (whole-wheat, low-sodium)

• 1/2 teaspoon black pepper freshly ground

• 2 teaspoons oregano , dry

• 2 tablespoons fresh basil leaves picked, then cut into thin strips or shredded

• 1/2 onion minced

• 1/2 cup egg beaters

Instructions

• Preheat oven to 350° F.

• In a large bowl, mix all ingredients together. Mold into 12 balls.

• Place balls on a nonstick baking sheet. Bake for 25 minutes.

Ingredients

- 1/2 cup fresh garlic minced

- yellow onion chopped

- 1 whole cabbage finely sliced, core cut out

- bay leaves

- 1/2 Tbsp basil (dry)

- 1/2 Tbsp oregano , dry

- 1 cup tomato puree (low sodium)

- 1 quart vegetable stock (low-sodium)

- 1/4 cup white vinegar

- 1/4 pound sugar cane stalks split

- 1 Tbsp Pritikin® All-Purpose Seasoning*

- 1 quart water

- 1/2 Tbsp coriander freshly ground

- 1 tsp black pepper freshly ground

Instructions

• In a large stock pot, saute garlic, onion, and cabbage on medium-high heat until onions are translucent, about 5 minutes.

• Add bay leaves, basil, oregano, tomato puree, vegetable stock, vinegar, sugar cane, Pritikin All-Purpose Seasoning, and water. Bring to boil, then simmer for 1 hour.

• Add coriander and black pepper. Remove sugar cane. Adjust vinegar and seasonings, if needed. Cook for 5 minutes more. Serve.

Potato Salad

Ingredients

• 3 pounds red bliss potatoes partially peeled

• 1 cup corn flakes fat free/no salt added

• 1/4 cup yogurt fat free

• 1/2 cup dill picked & chopped

• 1/2 teaspoon black peppercorns ground

• 1 teaspoon Splenda

- 1/4 cup cider vinegar

- 1 teaspoon Dijon mustard

- 1 tablespoon mustard (salt free stoneground)

Instructions

- Steam or boil potatoes until soft

- Mix remaining ingredients until well combined

- When Potatoes cool add dressing and let sit for at least 1 hour before serving

Conclusions

While high fat diets may promote short-term weight loss, the potential hazards for worsening risk for progression of atherosclerosis override the short-term benefits. Individuals derive the greatest health benefits from diets low in saturated fat and high in carbohydrate and fiber; these increase sensitivity to insulin and lower risk for CHD. Special diets are mainly used for unspecific health reasons by those who are females, have a college degree or with depression, and commonly used in conjunction with herbs and dietary supplements.

www.ingramcontent.com/pod-product-compliance
Lightning Source LLC
Chambersburg PA
CBHW070818170726
48000CB00018B/1321